GREEN GOODNESS

The Ultimate Guide To Enjoying A Greener Life

KARRY WILSON

ISBN: 9798863816272

\

Contents

INTRODUCTION

In today's fast-paced world, the quest for a vibrant and fulfilling life has led us to a profound appreciation of the power of nourishment. Beyond the age-old aspirations of shedding excess pounds and achieving overall well-being, the allure of embracing a wholesome diet stretches far beyond the conventional. In this digital age, a treasure trove of knowledge awaits those ready to embark on a journey towards healthier living. Let's unveil the multifaceted benefits of embracing a nourishing diet in the pursuit of a more vibrant and fulfilling life.

CHAPTER 1

The Modern Guide to Healthy Living

In the era of constant connectivity and evolving lifestyles, the significance of adopting a healthier diet transcends the conventional wisdom of yesteryears.

Beyond the well-known rewards of shedding unwanted weight and achieving general well-being, the benefits of embracing a nourishing diet in today's world are manifold.

Let's explore these advantages, backed by science and tailored to the demands of contemporary life.

The Fundamentals

Embracing a healthy diet is your key to sustainable weight management. No more starving yourself or relying on miracle pills.

By prioritizing nutritious foods, you can savor meals while still achieving your desired weight goals.

Your Ultimate Pharmacy

Did you know that what you eat can be your most potent defense against disease?

In an age where health conditions abound, it's crucial to acknowledge that many ailments stem from poor dietary choices.

Whether it's the excess fat and calories contributing to obesity, the lack of essential nutrients compromising your immune system, or the barrage of chemicals and trans fats in processed foods, unhealthy eating can have dire consequences for your well-being.

Revitalize Your Energy

Modern life demands high energy levels, and a balanced diet is your fuel. Unprocessed, whole foods are your allies, offering a wealth of nutrients.

When you nourish your body with fresh vegetables, lean proteins, and whole grains, you'll feel the surge of energy, enhancing your productivity and sociability.

Unlock Youthful Radiance

It's not just about feeling great; it's also about looking younger.

A nutritious diet promotes healthy cell growth, combatting free radicals and toxins in your body. Say hello to radiant skin and a youthful glow.

Boost Your Career

Healthy eating extends its benefits to your professional life. The discipline you cultivate in your diet can spill over into your work habits, making you more efficient and focused. Imagine the satisfaction of submitting your projects early, impressing your superiors, and perhaps even earning that long-awaited promotion.

Invest in Your Future

Your journey towards a healthier lifestyle can also translate into significant savings on healthcare costs. As insurance premiums continue to rise, safeguarding your health becomes an investment in reducing future medical expenses. By choosing wellness today, you're securing a healthier and more prosperous tomorrow.

CHAPTER 2

Unveiling the Wonders of Wheatgrass

In our quest for a healthier and more vibrant life, we delve into the verdant world of wheatgrass, a superfood with remarkable potential to elevate our well-being. In this chapter, we'll explore the myriad benefits of wheatgrass, shedding light on its modern applications and scientific insights.

The Red Blood-Cell Revolution

Wheatgrass emerges as a formidable ally in our pursuit of vitality. It has been scientifically proven to boost red blood cell count and lower blood pressure.

Its cleansing properties extend beyond mere detoxification; it purifies the bloodstream, vital organs, and gastrointestinal tract, ridding them of unwanted debris.

Daily consumption of wheatgrass juice invigorates metabolism and enhances the body's enzyme systems by enriching the blood. Moreover, it aids in reducing blood pressure by dilating blood vessels throughout the body.

A Potent Friend for Modern Ailments

The regular intake of wheatgrass juice, a popular means of reaping its nutritional benefits, can significantly benefit thyroid function. This, in turn, helps address contemporary health concerns such as obesity, indigestion, and a host of other common complaints.

Balancing the Body's Alkalinity

Wheatgrass juice acts as a natural balancer, restoring alkalinity to the blood. Abundant in alkaline minerals, it counters excessive acidity in the bloodstream.

Its versatility shines as it provides relief for various internal discomforts, effectively treating conditions like peptic ulcers, ulcerative inflammatory bowel disease, constipation, diarrhea, and other gastrointestinal issues.

The Ultimate Detoxifier

Among its many virtues, wheatgrass shines as a powerful detoxifier, offering crucial protection for the liver and blood. Packed with enzymes and amino acids, it stands alone in its ability to shield us from carcinogens, surpassing all other foods or medicines. It fortifies our cells, detoxifies our liver and bloodstream, and chemically neutralizes environmental pollutants.

A Guardian Against Tumors and Toxins

Recent research has unveiled wheatgrass juice's remarkable ability to combat tumors without the toxic side effects associated with conventional drugs that also target cell-destroying agents. The array of active compounds in wheatgrass juice cleanses the blood, neutralizes toxins, and facilitates their elimination from our cells.

Harnessing the Power of Enzymes

Enzymes are the unsung heroes of our health, and wheatgrass juice boasts an abundance of these vital catalysts. Whether you seek faster wound healing or desire weight loss, enzymes are at the heart of the process.

By introducing exogenous enzymes, such as those found in wheatgrass juice, we can extend the capabilities of the enzymes naturally present in our bodies. It's important to note that cooking wheatgrass destroys its enzyme content, so the full benefits are reaped when consumed raw.

Nature's Blueprint for Wellness

The nutritional profile of freshly juiced wheatgrass remarkably mirrors our own blood composition. Furthermore, chlorophyll, a key component of wheatgrass, bears a striking resemblance to hemoglobin, the molecule responsible for transporting oxygen in our blood.

This uncanny resemblance suggests that the "blood" of plants, when absorbed by humans, transforms into human blood, effectively distributing nutrients to every cell in our body.

In a world where health and vitality are paramount, wheatgrass emerges as a contemporary elixir, offering us a natural and powerful means to enrich our lives.

CHAPTER 3

The Power of Sprouts: A Modern Perspective on Health

In the ever-evolving landscape of nutrition and wellness, sprouts have emerged as a dynamic force, offering an array of health benefits. Let's explore the contemporary significance of sprouts and their role in promoting our well-being.

Discovering the Magic of Sprouts

Sprouts have captured the attention of health enthusiasts for their remarkable attributes. These tiny powerhouses are packed with essential nutrients and deserve a closer look in our quest for a healthier lifestyle.

A Legacy from the Roaring Twenties

Nearly a century ago, a forward-thinking professor introduced the concept of Bio-genic nutrition, heralding sprouted seeds and baby greens as the pinnacle of healthful foods.

He boldly suggested that these life-generating Bio-genic foods should constitute a quarter of our daily dietary intake, emphasizing their pivotal role in supporting cell regeneration.

The Battle Against Free Radicals

Various factors trigger the formation of free radicals within our bodies. These unstable oxygen molecules desperately seek electrons to stabilize their chaotic state.

In their quest, they pilfer electrons from healthy cells, resulting in the deterioration of vital biological structures and the alteration of DNA and RNA—a process known as oxidation.

However, superfoods like sprouts provide a robust source of antioxidants, comprising essential minerals, vitamins, and enzymes, which act as guardians against this damage.

The Alkaline Advantage

A healthy body thrives in an alkaline environment, devoid of excessive acidity. Bio-genic foods wield the power to alkalize the body, promoting balance and overall well-being. Raw foods, including sprouts, are oxygen-rich, and consistent consumption of these bio-genic wonders can be a boon to our health.

Oxygen, Alkalinity, and Disease

Research has unveiled the connection between a lack of oxygen and the growth of cancer cells, as well as the survival of viruses and bacteria. These entities struggle to thrive in an alkaline and oxygen-rich environment, highlighting the importance of incorporating bio-genic foods into our diets.

Fatty Acids and Immune Defense

Bio-genic foods are a potent source of crucial fatty acids—a nutrient often deficient in the typical Western diet. These fatty acids play a pivotal role in bolstering our immune system defenses, making sprouts an invaluable addition to our nutritional repertoire.

A Fiber-Rich Bounty

Sprouts are among the highest food sources of fiber, offering not only digestive benefits but also supporting overall gut health. A fiber-rich diet has a positive impact on various bodily functions, making it an essential component of a modern healthy lifestyle.

Unlocking Nutrient Potential

As sprouts grow and reach the chlorophyll-rich two-leaf stage, their nutritional profile undergoes a transformation. This transformation enhances the availability of vitamins, particularly B complex and C, in these tiny nutritional powerhouses.

Sprout biochemistry alters the mineral composition, making them more easily absorbed by the body. Additionally, it denatures protein into amino acid building blocks, facilitating digestion in half the time compared to cooked foods.

The significance of sprouts in promoting health and vitality cannot be overstated. These miniature marvels offer a holistic approach to wellness, enriching our lives with their nutritional abundance and potential.

CHAPTER 4

Juicing's Potential for Modern Health

In the hustle and bustle of contemporary life, we often find ourselves grappling with inadequate nutrition and an imbalance in our diets. Enter the rejuvenating world of juicing—a practice that not only modernizes our approach to consuming vegetables but also empowers us to attain optimal well-being.

Reviving Micronutrients through Juicing

In the realm of modern nutrition, cooking and processing have long been accused of stripping our food of essential micronutrients by altering their shape and chemical composition.

It's a lamentable truth that many of us fail to meet the recommended 6-8 servings of fruits and vegetables per day. The solution? Juicing—your passport to effortlessly achieving your daily veggie target.

The Fruit Factor: A Word of Caution

While juicing fruits may seem tempting, it's advisable to exercise caution, especially if you're dealing with weight issues, high blood pressure, diabetes, or elevated cholesterol levels.

However, lemons and limes emerge as exceptions to this rule, containing minimal damaging sugars like fructose. Additionally, these citrus wonders excel at neutralizing the bitterness often associated with dark leafy greens—the real heroes of juicing.

The Threefold Benefits of Veggie Juicing

Juicing offers a trifecta of advantages that modern health-conscious individuals can't afford to ignore:

Enhanced Nutrient Absorption: Over the years, many of us have compromised our digestion due to suboptimal food choices.

Juicing acts as a "pre-digestive" aid, ensuring that we absorb the maximum nutrition from our vegetables, preventing it from going to waste.

Efficient Veggie Consumption: For those who struggle to meet their daily vegetable intake, juicing provides an efficient solution. Tailored to your body weight, a glass of vegetable juice can help you meet your daily requirements with ease.

Diverse Nutritional Spectrum: Repetitive consumption of the same salads can lead to food allergies. With juicing, you can diversify your vegetable intake, introducing a broader range of nutrients that you might not typically enjoy whole.

Selecting the Right Veggies

If you're new to juicing, it's prudent to begin with pesticide-free or organic vegetables whenever possible. Some vegetables are more pesticide-laden than others, so exercise caution. Start with easily digestible options like celery, fennel, and cucumbers.

As you become accustomed to juicing, gradually introduce nutritionally dense but less palatable options like kale and collard greens.

Boosting Flavor and Health Benefits

To make your juice more palatable, consider adding components like lemon or lime (with the white rind intact), cranberries (in moderation), or even a dash of fresh ginger for that extra "kick." Researchers have even suggested that ginger may have a profound impact on cardiovascular health.

The Importance of Freshness

Juice is highly perishable, so it's crucial to consume it immediately or store it meticulously to prevent spoilage. Although many opt to juice in the morning, choose a mealtime that aligns with your lifestyle.

Cleanliness Is Key

After you've enjoyed your fresh juice, promptly clean your juicer to prevent mold growth and maintain its efficiency.

In the modern pursuit of health and vitality, juicing stands as an invaluable ally. With its power to revive and refresh our nutritional intake, juicing serves as a testament to our commitment to a vibrant and nourishing lifestyle.

CHAPTER 5

The Modern Era of Organics: Making Informed Choices

In today's ever-evolving food landscape, the once-exclusive realm of organic products has found its place on the shelves of mainstream supermarkets, posing a thoughtful dilemma for shoppers navigating the produce aisle. Picture this: a conventionally grown apple on one side and its organic counterpart on the other.

Both apples sport the same crispness, shine with vibrant red hues, and deliver essential vitamins, fiber, and fat-free goodness, all while remaining free of sodium and cholesterol. The question looms: which one do you choose?

The Organic Equation: What You Should Know

Amid the array of choices, it's essential to decipher whether organic food is not only a safer option but also a more nutritious one.

The term "organic" goes beyond just a label; it encompasses the philosophy behind the way farmers cultivate and process agricultural products—ranging from fruits and vegetables to grains, dairy, and meat.

Organic agricultural practices prioritize soil and water conservation while minimizing pollution. Organic farmers steer clear of conventional methods like chemical fertilization, weed control, and disease prevention. Instead, they employ advanced techniques such as crop rotations, mulching, and the use of manure to manage weeds and maintain the health of their livestock.

To maintain transparency and quality, the U.S. Department of Agriculture (USDA) has established rigorous organic certification standards that govern the cultivation, handling, and processing of organic foods.

Cracking the Organic Code: Labels Matter

When you embark on your organic journey at the grocery store, keep an eye out for the USDA Organic label. This label signifies that the product adheres to the USDA's stringent guidelines for production and processing. Products can fall into several categories:

100 Percent Organic: These single-ingredient foods, such as fruits, vegetables, and eggs, must bear this label to convey their complete organic nature.

Organic: Foods labeled as "organic" must contain at least 95 percent organic ingredients.

Made with Organic Ingredients: Products consisting of a minimum of 70 percent organic components may state "made with organic ingredients" on the label but can't use the USDA Organic seal or the term "organic."

Less than 70 Percent Organic Ingredients: Products falling below this threshold can't employ the term "organic" or display the USDA Organic seal but may include organic ingredients in their ingredient lists.

Decoding "Natural" vs. "Organic"

It's crucial to distinguish between "natural" and "organic." Phrases like "all natural," "free-range," or "hormone-free" might grace food labels, but they should not be conflated with "organic." Only foods grown and processed according to USDA organic criteria earn the coveted organic designation.

Pesticides and the Organic Advantage

Conventional growers often resort to pesticides to safeguard their crops against molds, insects, and diseases, leaving residual traces on produce. Concerns over pesticide residues have prompted some individuals to opt for organic food.

According to the USDA, organic produce typically contains significantly fewer pesticide residues compared to conventional counterparts. However, it's crucial to note that residues on most products—both organic and nonorganic—remain within government-established safety thresholds.

Nutrition Debate: Organic vs. Conventional

A recent comprehensive study reviewed scientific articles spanning five decades to scrutinize the nutrient content of organic and conventional foods. The verdict? Organically and conventionally produced foods exhibit strikingly similar nutrient profiles.

Ongoing research continues to shed light on this topic, underscoring the need for informed decision-making.

In the contemporary world of nutrition, the choice between conventional and organic foods is far from clear-cut. By understanding the nuances of organic labeling and the ongoing research in the field, you can navigate the aisles with confidence and make choices that align with your values and health priorities.

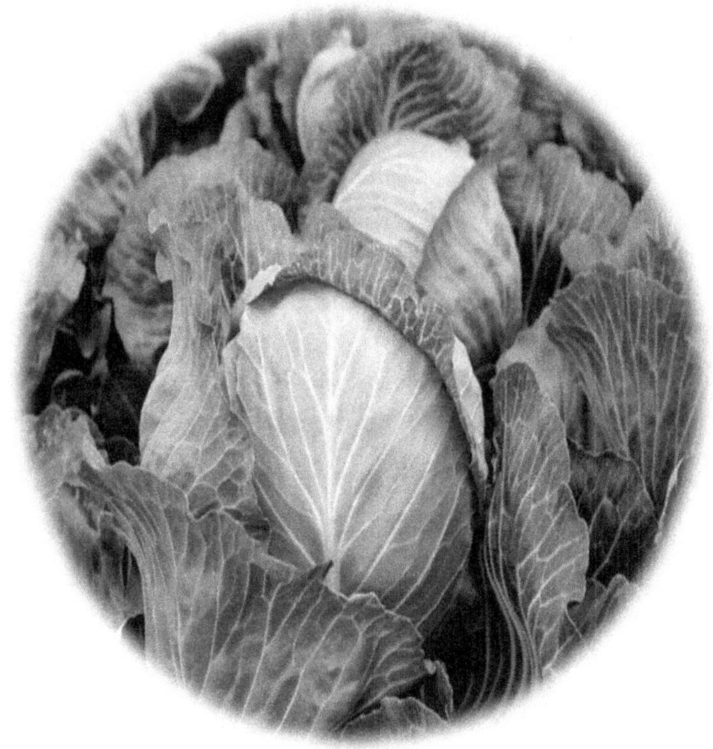

CHAPTER 6

Unveiling the Perils of Unhealthy Eating in the Modern Age

The choices we make about our diet have far-reaching consequences, influencing our well-being and longevity.

A healthy diet is not merely a buzzword but a powerful tool in fortifying our immune system, reducing the risk of illnesses, and enhancing our overall quality of life.

However, when years of unhealthy eating accumulate, these advantages can erode, leaving us vulnerable to severe conditions such as osteoporosis, hypertension, and cardiovascular diseases.

To safeguard our health and prevent these ailments, it is imperative to embrace a balanced, nutrient-rich diet long before the symptoms rear their heads.

The Health Gambit: Unmasking the Culprits

Osteoporosis, characterized by brittle bones that are highly susceptible to fractures, is often associated with advanced age, but its roots can be traced back to a lifetime of subpar nutrition.

As early as the twenties, especially in the case of women, calcium begins a gradual depletion from our bones.

Inadequate intake of calcium, vitamin D, and vitamin C, coupled with persistently low body weight, significantly heightens the risk of developing osteoporosis.

To mitigate the risk of osteoporosis, it is crucial to incorporate a diverse range of calcium-rich foods into our regular diets.

These include low-fat dairy products, calcium-fortified breads and grains, fortified juices and soy milk, as well as natural sources like spinach, salmon, sardines, and tofu.

Furthermore, vitamin C can be sourced from citrus fruits, tomatoes, and strawberries, while vitamin D can be obtained by spending short periods in the sun daily or through fortified dairy or soy products.

Hypertension: Breaking the Silent Threat

Hypertension, or high blood pressure, emerges when our arteries become clogged with plaque, a buildup that accumulates over time. Most of this arterial plaque is dietary in origin, often stemming from saturated fats, trans fats, excessive dietary cholesterol, and overconsumption in general.

Alarmingly, experts estimate that nearly half of all adults in America are at risk of developing hypertension, significantly increasing their chances of suffering a stroke, renal failure, heart attack, or heart failure.

Risk factors for hypertension include being overweight or obese, excessive sodium intake, insufficient potassium or vitamin D consumption, and excessive alcohol consumption.

To prevent or mitigate hypertension, it is advisable to cultivate a diet rich in a diverse array of healthy foods such as fruits, vegetables, whole grains, and lean protein sources. Reducing added sugars, saturated fats, and fried foods can further contribute to maintaining healthy blood pressure.

Regular physical activity is yet another effective means of preventing hypertension.

Guarding Against Cardiovascular Catastrophe

Cardiovascular diseases, encompassing heart disease, arteriosclerosis, congestive heart failure, heart attacks, and strokes, are formidable adversaries, often stemming from years of unwholesome eating habits.

A healthy diet emerges as one of the most potent weapons in our arsenal against these life-threatening conditions.

Foods laden with saturated fats (common in fatty meats, cheese, butter, and eggs) and trans fats (found in shortening, margarine, fried and processed snacks) escalate the risk of cardiovascular diseases. In contrast, nutrient-rich foods like fruits, vegetables, whole grains, legumes, and lean protein sources can serve as potent allies in reducing this risk.

Additionally, incorporating at least two servings of fatty fish such as salmon, tuna, or mackerel each week can supply the body with omega-3 fatty acids, heart-healthy fats that are essential for maintaining cardiovascular health.

In our ongoing quest for long-term well-being and the prevention of diet-related diseases, it is incumbent upon us to adopt a balanced diet, replete with a wide spectrum of nutritious foods.

This modern approach to nutrition offers us the power to chart a course towards a healthier, more vibrant future.

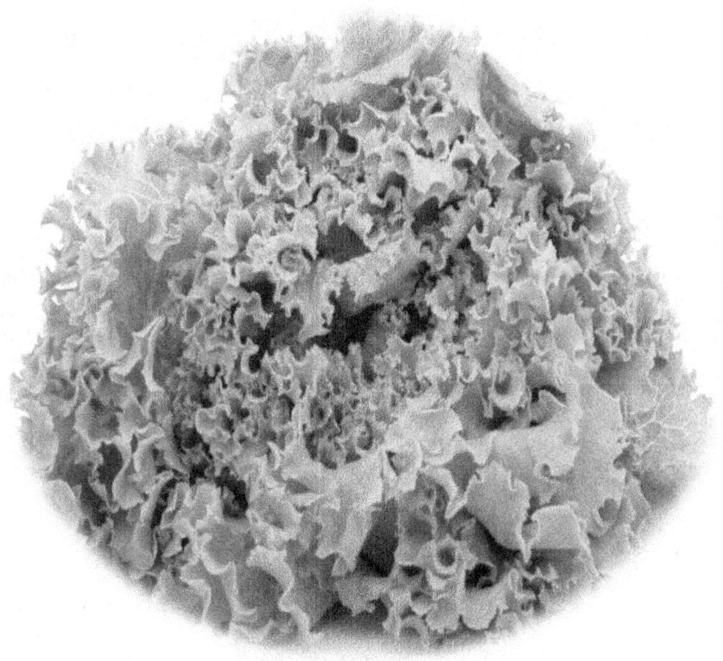

CHAPTER 7

Unleashing the Power of Superfoods

In an era where health-conscious choices and holistic well-being have taken center stage, superfoods have emerged as the nutritional heroes of our time. These remarkable foods, often celebrated for their exceptional nutrient density and health benefits, have become the darlings of the culinary world and the focal point of many health-conscious diets.

Let's embark on a journey into the fascinating realm of superfoods, where we'll uncover the secrets behind their nutritional prowess and learn how to harness their potential to transform our diets and elevate our overall health.

Defining Superfoods: Nutritional Powerhouses

Superfoods, by definition, are foods that are exceptionally rich in essential nutrients, vitamins, minerals, and antioxidants. These nutritional powerhouses go above and beyond typical dietary staples, offering a concentrated dose of health benefits in every bite. Superfoods come in various forms, ranging from fruits and vegetables to grains, nuts, and seeds, each with its unique set of nutrients and wellness perks.

The Magic of Antioxidants

One of the standout features of many superfoods is their high antioxidant content. Antioxidants are compounds that help protect our bodies from oxidative stress and free radicals—unstable molecules that can damage our cells and contribute to chronic diseases, including cancer and heart disease.

Superfoods like blueberries, kale, and dark chocolate are celebrated for their potent antioxidant properties, making them essential additions to any health-conscious diet.

Nutrient Density: Quality Over Quantity

Superfoods are synonymous with nutrient density, a concept that emphasizes the quality of nutrients in a food item rather than its quantity.

This means that superfoods provide a substantial amount of essential nutrients, such as vitamins, minerals, and dietary fiber, while often being relatively low in calories. For individuals looking to maximize their nutritional intake without overindulging in calories, superfoods offer an ideal solution.

The Versatility of Superfoods

One of the most exciting aspects of superfoods is their versatility in the kitchen. From acai bowls to quinoa salads, superfoods can be seamlessly integrated into a wide range of dishes, catering to various tastes and culinary preferences.

Whether you're a fan of savory or sweet, there's a superfood for every palate.

The Superfood Lineup

The world of superfoods is vast and diverse, with each food item bringing its unique set of health benefits to the table. Here are just a few superstars in the superfood lineup:

Berries: Blueberries, strawberries, and acai berries are bursting with antioxidants and vitamins, making them excellent choices for boosting immunity and promoting radiant skin.

Leafy Greens: Spinach, kale, and Swiss chard are packed with vitamins, minerals, and fiber, offering support for bone health and overall vitality.

Nuts and Seeds: Almonds, chia seeds, and flaxseeds are rich in heart-healthy fats, fiber, and protein, making them essential for a well-rounded diet.

Fatty Fish: Salmon, mackerel, and sardines provide omega-3 fatty acids, known for their anti-inflammatory properties and their positive impact on heart health.

Turmeric: This vibrant spice contains curcumin, a powerful anti-inflammatory compound associated with a range of health benefits, including improved joint health and cognitive function.

Incorporating Superfoods into Your Diet

Adding superfoods to your daily meals can be a delightful and rewarding experience. Whether you choose to sprinkle chia seeds on your morning yogurt, blend kale into your daily smoothie, or indulge in a square of dark chocolate after dinner, there are countless ways to incorporate these nutritional gems into your diet.

Superfoods can complement a variety of dietary preferences, including vegan, vegetarian, and omnivorous diets, making them accessible to individuals with diverse culinary lifestyles.

By introducing superfoods into your diet, you can enhance your nutritional intake, boost your immune system, and take proactive steps toward long-term health and vitality.

The Future of Superfoods

As research continues to uncover the remarkable health benefits of superfoods, it's clear that these nutritional powerhouses will play a pivotal role in shaping the future of nutrition and wellness.

From supporting heart health to enhancing cognitive function, superfoods offer a promising path to a healthier and more vibrant life.

CHAPTER 8

The Art of Mindful Eating

In our fast-paced world, where the cacophony of daily life often drowns out the subtleties of our existence, the practice of mindful eating offers a profound opportunity to reconnect with the present moment and cultivate a deeper relationship with the food we consume.

This age-old concept, adapted for the modern era, invites us to savor each bite, appreciate the intricate flavors, and embrace the profound benefits of conscious consumption.

Join us as we delve into the art of mindful eating—a practice that not only enhances our relationship with food but also brings about better digestion and overall contentment.

The Lost Connection

In the rush of our daily lives, many of us have lost touch with the true essence of eating. We often find ourselves consuming meals hurriedly, multitasking during mealtimes, or mindlessly munching on snacks while distracted by screens or other stimuli.

This disconnection from our food and our bodies can lead to a host of issues, including overeating, digestive discomfort, and a lack of appreciation for the nourishment that sustains us.

What Is Mindful Eating?

At its core, mindful eating is the practice of bringing full awareness and attention to the act of eating. It involves being present in the moment, engaging all our senses, and savoring each bite with gratitude and curiosity.

Mindful eating encourages us to pay attention to not only what we eat but also how we eat it, fostering a deep appreciation for the food on our plates.

The Benefits of Mindful Eating

The benefits of mindful eating extend far beyond the dinner table. Here are some of the advantages that this practice can bring into your life:

Improved Digestion: When we eat mindfully, we give our bodies the time they need to digest food properly. This can alleviate common digestive issues like bloating, gas, and indigestion.

Better Relationship with Food: Mindful eating helps us break free from unhealthy eating patterns, such as emotional eating or binge eating. It encourages a balanced and harmonious relationship with food.

Enhanced Enjoyment: By savoring each bite and paying attention to flavors and textures, we derive more pleasure from our meals. Food becomes a source of joy and nourishment.

Weight Management: Mindful eating can aid in weight management by promoting a healthy awareness of hunger and fullness cues, preventing overeating.

Stress Reduction: This practice fosters a sense of calm and relaxation during meals, reducing stress and promoting overall well-being.

How to Practice Mindful Eating

Engage Your Senses: Begin by truly seeing, smelling, and appreciating your food. Observe its colors, textures, and aroma. Let your senses come alive.

Slow Down: Eat at a slower pace, taking the time to chew each bite thoroughly. Put your utensils down between bites to prevent rushing.

Eliminate Distractions: Turn off the TV, put away your phone, and create a calm and focused eating environment. Eating in silence or with pleasant background music can enhance the experience.

Listen to Your Body: Tune into your body's hunger and fullness cues. Eat when you're hungry and stop when you're satisfied, rather than following rigid meal times or portion sizes.

Appreciate Each Bite: Savor the flavors, textures, and sensations of your food. Try to identify the different ingredients and spices in your dish.

Practice Gratitude: Take a moment to express gratitude for the nourishment you're receiving. Reflect on the journey your food took to reach your plate.

Mindful Meal Planning: Extend mindfulness to meal planning and preparation. Choose whole, nourishing ingredients and cook with care and intention.

Beyond the Plate

The practice of mindful eating extends beyond what's on your plate. It encompasses an entire approach to life, promoting mindfulness in all aspects of daily living. By embracing mindfulness in our relationship with food, we unlock a pathway to a more harmonious and balanced existence.

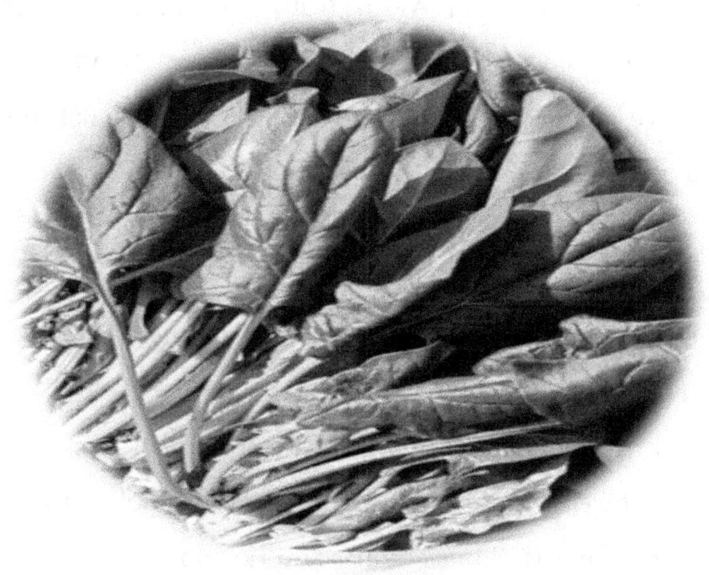

CHAPTER 9

The Digital Age of Nutrition

In the digital age, where technology has permeated every aspect of our lives, it's no surprise that nutrition is also undergoing a significant transformation. The convergence of smartphones, wearable devices, and online resources has ushered in a new era of dietary awareness and wellness.

Welcome to the Digital Age of Nutrition, where we explore the myriad ways in which technology is revolutionizing the way we approach our dietary choices, track our nutrition, and optimize our health.

The Rise of Nutrition Apps

Nutrition apps have become ubiquitous tools for individuals seeking to monitor and improve their dietary habits. These apps offer a convenient way to track daily food intake, count calories, and analyze the nutritional content of meals. Some popular nutrition apps even provide personalized meal plans and dietary recommendations based on individual goals and preferences.

Wearable Devices and Health Trackers

The integration of wearable devices into our daily lives has extended to the realm of nutrition and fitness. Smartwatches and fitness trackers can now monitor various health metrics, including heart rate, sleep patterns, and even calorie expenditure. These devices provide real-time feedback and encourage users to stay active and make healthier choices throughout the day.

Online Recipe Platforms

The internet has given rise to an abundance of online recipe platforms and cooking websites. These platforms offer a wealth of culinary inspiration, from quick and easy weekday recipes to gourmet dishes for special occasions.

Users can access a vast library of recipes, complete with step-by-step instructions and nutritional information, making it easier than ever to prepare wholesome and delicious meals at home.

Personalized Nutrition Plans

Advancements in artificial intelligence and machine learning have paved the way for personalized nutrition plans. By analyzing an individual's dietary preferences, health goals, and genetic factors, these algorithms can generate tailored meal plans and dietary recommendations.

This personalized approach to nutrition ensures that individuals receive dietary guidance that aligns with their unique needs.

Virtual Nutrition Coaches

Virtual nutrition coaches and dietitian services have gained popularity, offering users access to professional dietary guidance and support through online platforms.

These virtual coaches can provide expert advice, answer questions, and assist individuals in making informed dietary decisions. This accessibility allows for greater flexibility in seeking nutritional guidance.

The Importance of Data Privacy

While the Digital Age of Nutrition offers numerous benefits, it also raises concerns about data privacy and security.

As individuals share personal health information and dietary preferences on digital platforms, safeguarding this sensitive data becomes paramount. It is essential for users to be mindful of the privacy policies of nutrition apps and online platforms to protect their personal information.

Navigating the Digital Landscape

As we navigate the digital landscape of nutrition, it's crucial to strike a balance between technology and mindful eating.

While these digital tools offer valuable insights and convenience, they should complement our overall well-being rather than dominate it. It's essential to remember that technology is a tool, and the foundation of a healthy diet remains rooted in balanced food choices, portion control, and a mindful approach to eating.

The Digital Age of Nutrition is an exciting era that empowers individuals to take charge of their dietary health like never before.

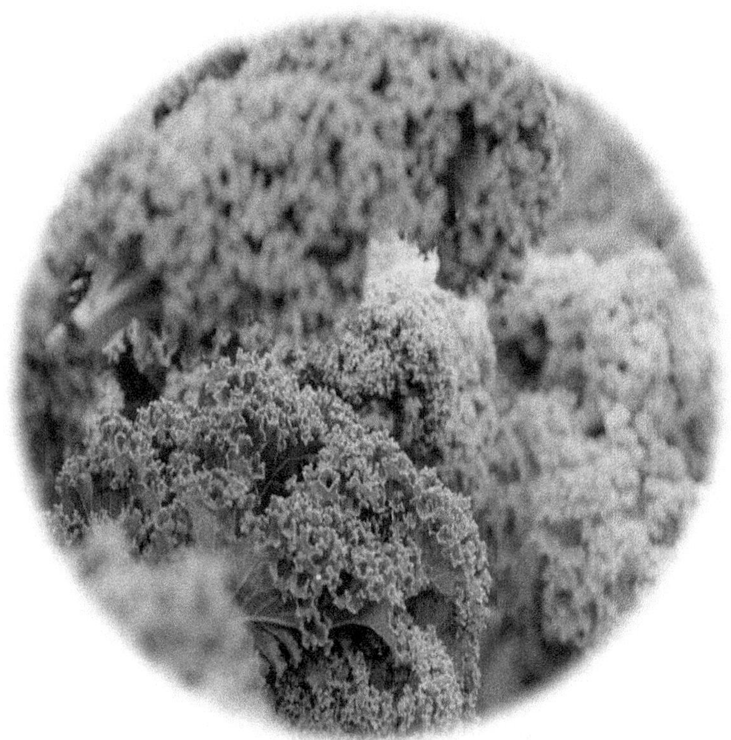

CHAPTER 10

The Future of Food: Sustainable and Plant-Based

As our world grapples with the challenges of climate change, resource scarcity, and a growing global population, the future of food is at a crossroads. The solution to many of these pressing issues lies in a shift towards sustainable and plant-based diets.

In this chapter, we explore the evolving landscape of food choices, emphasizing the vital role of sustainability and the rise of plant-based diets in shaping the future of our food.

The Imperative for Sustainability

Sustainability has emerged as a non-negotiable priority in the food industry.

The current methods of food production, including intensive livestock farming and monoculture crop cultivation, contribute significantly to greenhouse gas emissions, deforestation, and soil degradation.

The consequences of these practices are detrimental to both the environment and human health.

Sustainable food practices aim to mitigate these negative impacts by adopting eco-friendly methods of production, reducing waste, and promoting biodiversity.

This approach prioritizes the long-term well-being of our planet and future generations.

Plant-Based Diets: A Growing Movement

The plant-based diet movement is gaining momentum worldwide, driven by concerns about health, animal welfare, and the environment. Plant-based diets emphasize the consumption of foods derived from plants, such as fruits, vegetables, legumes, grains, nuts, and seeds, while minimizing or eliminating animal products.

This dietary shift offers several benefits:

Environmental Impact: Plant-based diets have a significantly lower carbon footprint compared to traditional meat-heavy diets. They require fewer natural resources, produce fewer greenhouse gas emissions, and reduce deforestation associated with livestock farming.

Health Benefits: Plant-based diets are associated with lower rates of chronic diseases, including heart disease, diabetes, and certain types of cancer. They are typically lower in saturated fats and cholesterol while being rich in fiber, vitamins, and antioxidants.

Animal Welfare: Choosing plant-based options aligns with ethical concerns about animal welfare. It reduces demand for factory farming and the suffering of animals raised for food.

Food Security: Plant-based diets can enhance global food security by utilizing resources more efficiently. With the world's population expected to reach 9 billion by 2050, sustainable food production is paramount.

The Role of Food Technology

The future of food is intertwined with advancements in food technology. Innovations in plant-based alternatives to traditional animal products are reshaping the market.

Plant-based burgers that mimic the taste and texture of beef, dairy-free milk, and vegan cheese are just a few examples of how technology is transforming the plant-based landscape.

Additionally, sustainable agriculture practices, such as vertical farming, aquaponics, and precision agriculture, are emerging as solutions to increase food production while minimizing resource use.

Embracing a Sustainable Future

To secure a sustainable and plant-based future of food, individuals, businesses, and policymakers must take action:

Consumer Choices: As consumers, we can make mindful choices by reducing our meat consumption, supporting local and sustainable agriculture, and opting for plant-based alternatives.

Business Initiatives: Food companies have a pivotal role to play by investing in research and development of sustainable and plant-based products, reducing food waste, and adopting eco-friendly packaging.

Policy Changes: Governments can implement policies that incentivize sustainable farming practices, reduce subsidies for unsustainable agriculture, and promote dietary guidelines that prioritize plant-based options.

Education and Awareness: Raising awareness about the environmental and health impacts of dietary choices is essential. Educational programs and campaigns can inform the public about the benefits of sustainable and plant-based diets.

The future of food is not just a matter of personal choice; it is a global imperative. By embracing sustainability and adopting plant-based diets, we can pave the way for a more resilient, ethical, and nourishing food system—one that nourishes both our bodies and our planet.

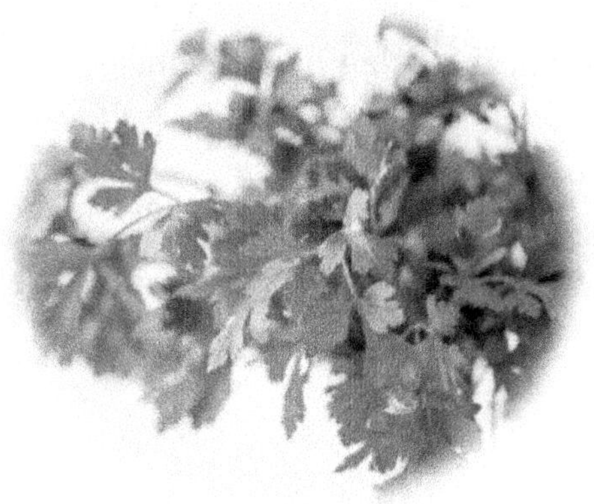

Conclusion

Nourishing Your Way to a Brighter Future

In the fast-paced, high-stress world we live in today, taking charge of your health through wise dietary choices is more crucial than ever. It's not just about shedding a few pounds or looking good; it's about nurturing your body and mind to thrive in the face of life's challenges.

By fueling your body with the right nutrients and practicing mindful eating, you're not only reducing the detrimental effects of stress but also enhancing your overall well-being. Stress is an inevitable part of life, but how you respond to it can make all the difference.

Think of your health as an investment—an investment in a future where you're not only living longer but also living better. The benefits of a healthy diet extend far beyond physical appearance; they encompass mental clarity, emotional resilience, and a zest for life that knows no bounds.

As you prioritize your health and make informed choices about what you put on your plate, remember that you're not just improving your present; you're securing a brighter, more vibrant future. The increased vitality and productivity you experience today will pay off in dividends as you chart the course for the years ahead.

So, embrace the power of healthy eating, and let it propel you towards a life of boundless possibilities. Your health is your greatest asset, and by nourishing it with wholesome foods, you're nourishing the remarkable journey that lies ahead.